MIND DIET SMOOTHIE RECIPES COOKBOOK

Delicious and Nutritious Recipes for Brain Health, Alzheimer's and to Boost Cognitive Wellness

By

Dr. Donna Matias

Table of Contents

Introduction to the MIND Diet

Welcome to the MIND Diet Smoothie Recipes Cookbook! In this guide, we embark on a journey to explore the intersection of nutrition and cognitive wellness. The MIND diet, which stands for the Mediterranean-DASH Intervention for Neurodegenerative Delay, is a dietary pattern specifically designed to support brain health and reduce the risk of cognitive decline.

As we navigate through the pages of this cookbook, we'll delve into the rich world of smoothies—a delicious and convenient way to incorporate the key principles of the MIND diet into your daily routine. Each recipe has been carefully crafted to feature ingredients known for their brain-boosting properties, from vibrant berries and leafy greens to healthy fats and antioxidant-rich spices.

But this cookbook is more than just a collection of recipes; it's a comprehensive guide to nourishing your brain through mindful eating. In addition to tantalizing smoothie creations, you'll find essential tips for creating the perfect blend, insights into the nutritional science behind each ingredient, and practical advice for incorporating smoothies into your lifestyle.

Whether you're seeking to support cognitive function, enhance mental clarity, or simply enjoy delicious and nutritious beverages, the MIND Diet Smoothie Recipes Cookbook is your go-to resource. Join us on this culinary journey as we harness the power of food to nourish our minds and cultivate a lifetime of cognitive wellness.

Understanding the MIND Diet

Importance of Nutrition for Brain Health

Nutrition plays a fundamental role in maintaining optimal brain health throughout life. Just as our bodies require nourishment to function efficiently, our brains also depend on a steady supply of nutrients to support cognitive function, memory, mood regulation, and overall mental well-being. Here are some key reasons why nutrition is crucial for brain health:

- **Fueling Brain Function:** The brain is one of the most metabolically active organs in the body, requiring a constant supply of energy to carry out its myriad functions. Glucose, derived from carbohydrates in the diet, is the primary source of fuel for the brain. Adequate intake of carbohydrates ensures that the brain receives the energy it needs to perform tasks ranging from basic physiological functions to complex cognitive processes.

- **Providing Essential Nutrients:** Essential nutrients, including vitamins, minerals, antioxidants, and fatty acids, play vital roles in brain health. For example, omega-3 fatty acids found in fatty fish, flaxseeds, and walnuts are important for brain development, cognitive function, and mood regulation. Antioxidants such as vitamin C, vitamin E, and polyphenols help protect brain cells from oxidative stress and inflammation, which are implicated in neurodegenerative diseases and cognitive decline.

- **Supporting Neurotransmitter Production:** Neurotransmitters are chemical messengers that facilitate communication between brain cells (neurons) and regulate various physiological processes, including mood, sleep, and cognition. Certain nutrients, such as amino acids from protein-rich foods, are precursors to neurotransmitters like serotonin, dopamine, and acetylcholine. A balanced diet that includes adequate protein helps ensure optimal neurotransmitter synthesis, promoting mental clarity and emotional well-being.

- **Promoting Brain Plasticity:** Brain plasticity, also known as neuroplasticity, refers to the brain's ability to adapt and reorganize in response to experiences, learning, and environmental influences. Nutrition plays a critical role in supporting brain plasticity by providing the building blocks necessary for the formation of new neural connections and the repair of damaged neurons. Nutrients like choline, found in eggs and leafy greens, and phospholipids, abundant in nuts and seeds, are essential for maintaining the structural integrity of cell membranes and facilitating communication between neurons.

• **Reducing Risk of Cognitive Decline:** Mounting evidence suggests that certain dietary patterns, such as the Mediterranean-style diet and the MIND diet, are associated with a reduced risk of cognitive decline and neurodegenerative diseases like Alzheimer's disease. These diets prioritize whole foods rich in fruits, vegetables, whole grains, lean proteins, and healthy fats, while minimizing intake of processed foods, sugary snacks, and saturated fats. By adopting a brain-healthy diet, individuals can potentially mitigate risk factors for cognitive decline and optimize brain function throughout the lifespan.

The Power of Smoothies for Cognitive Wellness

Smoothies have emerged as a popular and convenient way to pack a nutritional punch into one delicious and refreshing beverage. Beyond their taste and convenience, smoothies offer a multitude of benefits for cognitive wellness. Here's how smoothies can support brain health and promote cognitive function:

• **Nutrient Density:** Smoothies provide an easy and efficient way to incorporate a variety of nutrient-rich ingredients into one serving. By blending together fruits, vegetables, nuts, seeds, and other brain-boosting foods, smoothies deliver a diverse array of vitamins, minerals, antioxidants, and phytonutrients that support cognitive function and overall brain health. Consuming a nutrient-dense smoothie can help ensure that your brain receives the essential nutrients it needs to thrive.

- **Hydration:** Proper hydration is crucial for maintaining optimal brain function. Dehydration can impair cognitive performance, leading to symptoms such as decreased concentration, fatigue, and brain fog. Smoothies offer a hydrating option, especially when made with hydrating ingredients like water-rich fruits (e.g., watermelon, cucumber) and coconut water. Staying hydrated throughout the day can help support cognitive wellness and mental clarity.

• **Blood Sugar Regulation:** Fluctuations in blood sugar levels can impact cognitive function and mood. Consuming foods with a high glycemic index, such as sugary snacks and refined carbohydrates, can lead to spikes and crashes in blood sugar levels, contributing to cognitive impairment and mood swings. Smoothies that incorporate fiber-rich fruits, vegetables, and healthy fats can help stabilize blood sugar levels, providing a steady source of energy to the brain and promoting cognitive stability.

• **Gut-Brain Connection:** Emerging research suggests a strong connection between the gut and the brain, known as the gut-brain axis. The gut microbiome, composed of trillions of microorganisms that inhabit the digestive tract, plays a crucial role in regulating brain function and mood. Certain ingredients commonly found in smoothies, such as probiotic-rich yogurt, fiber-rich fruits and vegetables, and prebiotic sources like oats and flaxseeds, can support a healthy gut microbiome, leading to improved cognitive wellness and mood regulation.

- **Convenience and Portability:** In today's fast-paced world, convenience is key when it comes to maintaining healthy eating habits. Smoothies offer a portable and on-the-go option for nourishing your brain wherever you are. Whether you're rushing out the door in the morning or need a mid-afternoon pick-me-up, a nutrient-packed smoothie can provide a quick and convenient way to fuel your brain and support cognitive function throughout the day.

Incorporating smoothies into your daily routine can be a delicious and effective strategy for promoting cognitive wellness. By blending together a variety of brain-boosting ingredients, staying hydrated, stabilizing blood sugar levels, supporting gut health, and enjoying the convenience of a portable meal or snack, you can harness the power of smoothies to nourish your brain and optimize cognitive function.

Benefits of Smoothies for Brain Health

Smoothies have garnered attention as a convenient and delicious way to nourish the body, but their benefits extend beyond mere refreshment—they can significantly support brain health. Here are several ways in which smoothies contribute to optimal cognitive function and overall brain health:

- **Nutrient-Rich Ingredients:** Smoothies offer a versatile platform to incorporate a wide variety of nutrient-rich ingredients, including fruits, vegetables, nuts, seeds, and superfoods. These ingredients are abundant in vitamins, minerals, antioxidants, and phytonutrients, which play crucial roles in brain health. For example, berries are rich in flavonoids, which have been linked to improved cognitive function, while leafy greens provide essential vitamins and minerals that support overall brain health.

- **Antioxidant Protection:** Many ingredients commonly used in smoothies, such as berries, spinach, kale, and nuts, are rich in antioxidants. Antioxidants help neutralize harmful free radicals in the body, reducing oxidative stress and inflammation that can damage brain cells and contribute to cognitive decline. Regular consumption of antioxidant-rich smoothies may help protect against age-related neurodegenerative diseases, such as Alzheimer's and Parkinson's disease.

- **Healthy Fats:** Smoothies can be an excellent source of healthy fats, which are essential for brain health. Ingredients like avocados, nuts, seeds, and nut butters provide omega-3 and omega-6 fatty acids, which support brain structure and function. These fats are crucial for maintaining the integrity of cell membranes, facilitating communication between brain cells, and promoting the formation of new neural connections, all of which are essential for optimal cognitive function.

- **Blood Sugar Regulation:** The ingredients used in smoothies, particularly when combined with protein and healthy fats, can help stabilize blood sugar levels. Fluctuations in blood sugar can negatively impact cognitive function and mood, leading to brain fog and fatigue. By including fiber-rich fruits, vegetables, and ingredients like protein powder or Greek yogurt, smoothies can help maintain steady blood sugar levels, providing a sustained source of energy to the brain.

• **Hydration:** Proper hydration is essential for brain health, as even mild dehydration can impair cognitive function and focus. Smoothies are an excellent way to boost hydration, especially when made with hydrating ingredients like water-rich fruits (e.g., watermelon, cucumber), coconut water, or herbal teas. Staying hydrated supports optimal brain function and can help improve memory, concentration, and mental clarity.

- **Gut-Brain Connection:** Emerging research highlights the importance of the gut-brain axis—the bidirectional communication between the gut and the brain—in regulating mood, cognition, and overall brain health. Smoothies that incorporate gut-friendly ingredients like probiotic-rich yogurt, prebiotic fibers, and fermented foods can support a healthy gut microbiome, which in turn positively influences brain function and mental well-being.

Berry Blends for Brain Boosting

Blueberry Brain Blast:

Ingredients:

- 1 cup blueberries (fresh or frozen)

- 1 ripe banana

- 1/2 cup spinach leaves

- 1/2 cup plain Greek yogurt

- 1 tablespoon almond butter

- 1/2 cup unsweetened almond milk

- Ice cubes (optional)

Preparation:

- Place all ingredients in a blender.

- Blend until smooth and creamy.

- If desired, add ice cubes and blend again until desired consistency is reached.

- Pour into a glass and enjoy!

Raspberry Antioxidant Delight:

Ingredients:

- 1 cup raspberries (fresh or frozen)

- 1/2 cup strawberries (fresh or frozen)

- 1/2 cup spinach leaves

- 1/2 cup plain Greek yogurt

- 1 tablespoon chia seeds

- 1/2 cup unsweetened almond milk

- Ice cubes (optional)

Preparation:

- Combine all ingredients in a blender.

- Blend until smooth and creamy.

- Add ice cubes if you desired and blend again until smooth.

- Pour into a glass and serve immediately.

Strawberry Spinach Sensation:

Ingredients:

- 1 cup strawberries (fresh or frozen)

- 1/2 cup spinach leaves

- 1/2 ripe avocado

- 1 tablespoon of honey or maple syrup. (optional)

- 1/2 cup coconut water

- Ice cubes (optional)

Preparation:

- In a blender, combine strawberries, spinach, avocado, and honey or maple syrup (if using).

- Add coconut water to the blender.

- Blend until smooth and creamy.

- If desired, add ice cubes and blend again until desired consistency is reached.

- Pour into a glass and serve immediately.

Blackberry Banana Bliss:

Ingredients:

- 1 cup blackberries (fresh or frozen)

- 1 ripe banana

- 1/2 cup plain Greek yogurt

- 1 tablespoon almond butter

- 1/2 cup unsweetened almond milk

- Ice cubes (optional)

Preparation:

- Place blackberries, banana, Greek yogurt, almond butter, and almond milk in a blender.

- Blend until smooth and creamy.

- Add ice cubes if you desired and blend again until smooth.

- Pour into a glass and enjoy!

Mixed Berry Powerhouse:

Ingredients:

- 1/2 cup strawberries (fresh or frozen)

- 1/2 cup blueberries (fresh or frozen)

- 1/2 cup raspberries (fresh or frozen)

- 1/2 cup spinach leaves

- 1/2 cup plain Greek yogurt

- 1 tablespoon of honey or maple syrup. (optional)

- 1/2 cup water or coconut water

- Ice cubes (optional)

Preparation:

- Combine strawberries, blueberries, raspberries, spinach, Greek yogurt, honey or maple syrup (if using), and water or coconut water in a blender.

● Blend until smooth and creamy.

● If desired, add ice cubes and blend again until desired consistency is reached.

● Pour into a glass and serve immediately.

Cranberry Orange Brain Booster:

Ingredients:

● 1/2 cup cranberries (fresh or frozen)

● 1 orange, peeled and segmented

● 1/2 cup spinach leaves

- 1/2 cup plain Greek yogurt

- 1 tablespoon flaxseed meal

- 1/2 cup unsweetened almond milk

- Ice cubes (optional)

Preparation:

- In a blender, combine cranberries, orange segments, spinach, Greek yogurt, flaxseed meal, and almond milk.

- Blend until smooth and creamy.

- Add ice cubes if you desired and blend again until smooth.

- Pour into a glass and enjoy!

Acai Berry Brain Boost:

Ingredients:

- 1/2 cup frozen acai puree or acai berry powder

- 1/2 cup mixed berries (such as strawberries, blueberries, and raspberries)

- 1/2 ripe banana

- 1/2 cup spinach leaves

- 1/2 cup plain Greek yogurt

- 1 tablespoon honey or maple syrup (optional)

- 1/2 cup coconut water or your almond milk

- Ice cubes (optional)

Preparation:

• Combine acai puree or powder, mixed berries, banana, spinach, Greek yogurt, honey or maple syrup (if using), and coconut water or almond milk in a blender.

• Blend until smooth and creamy.

• Add ice cubes if you desired and blend again until smooth.

• Pour into a glass and serve immediately.

Goji Berry Brain Fuel:

Ingredients:

- 1/4 cup goji berries. (soaked in water for 10-15 minutes)

- 1/2 cup strawberries (fresh or frozen)

- 1/2 cup blueberries (fresh or frozen)

- 1/2 cup spinach leaves

- 1/2 cup plain Greek yogurt

- 1 tablespoon almond butter

- 1/2 cup unsweetened almond milk

- Ice cubes (optional)

Preparation:

- Drain the soaked goji berries and place them in a blender.

- Add strawberries, blueberries, spinach, Greek yogurt, almond butter, and almond milk to the blender.

- Blend until smooth and creamy.

- If desired, add ice cubes and blend again until desired consistency is reached.

- Pour into a glass and enjoy!

These smoothie recipes are packed with brain-boosting ingredients and are a delicious way to support cognitive function and overall brain health. Adjust the sweetness and consistency according to your preference and enjoy these nutrient-rich blends as part of a balanced diet.

Green Goodness for Cognitive Function

Spinach Avocado Elixir:

Ingredients:

- 1 cup spinach leaves

- 1/2 ripe avocado

- 1/2 cup pineapple chunks. (fresh or frozen)

- 1/2 cup plain Greek yogurt

- 1 tablespoon of honey or maple syrup. (optional)

- 1/2 cup coconut water or your almond milk

- Ice cubes (optional)

Preparation:

- Place spinach leaves, avocado, pineapple chunks, Greek yogurt, honey or maple syrup (if using), and coconut water or almond milk in a blender.

- Blend until smooth and creamy.

- Add ice cubes if you desired and blend again until desired consistency is reached.

- Pour into a glass and serve immediately.

Kale Pineapple Refresher:

Ingredients:

- 1 cup kale leaves, stems removed

- 1/2 cup pineapple chunks (fresh or frozen)

- 1/2 banana

- 1/2 cup coconut water or almond milk

- 1 tablespoon chia seeds

- Ice cubes (optional)

Preparation:

- Combine kale leaves, pineapple chunks, banana, coconut water or almond milk, and chia seeds in a blender.

- Blend until smooth and creamy.

- Add ice cubes if desired and blend again until smooth.

- Pour into a glass and enjoy!

Cucumber Mint Revitalizer:

Ingredients:

- 1 cucumber, peeled and chopped

- Handful of fresh mint leaves

- Juice of 1 lime

- 1 tablespoon honey or maple syrup (optional)

- 1/2 cup coconut water

- Ice cubes (optional)

Preparation:

- Place chopped cucumber, mint leaves, lime juice, honey or maple syrup (if using), and coconut water in a blender.

- Blend until smooth.

- Add ice cubes if desired and blend again until desired consistency is reached.

- Pour into a glass, garnish with mint leaves if desired, and serve immediately.

Matcha Mango Madness:

Ingredients:

- 1 teaspoon matcha powder

- 1/2 cup mango chunks (fresh or frozen)

- 1/2 banana

- 1/2 cup spinach leaves

- 1/2 cup plain Greek yogurt

- 1/2 cup unsweetened almond milk

- Ice cubes (optional)

Preparation:

- In a blender, combine matcha powder, mango chunks, banana, spinach leaves, Greek yogurt, and almond milk.

- Blend until smooth and creamy.

- Add ice cubes if you desired and blend again until smooth.

- Pour into a glass and enjoy this refreshing brain-boosting smoothie!

Kiwi Coconut Brain Booster:

Ingredients:

- 2 kiwis, peeled and sliced

- 1/2 cup coconut milk

- 1/2 cup spinach leaves

- 1 tablespoon honey or maple syrup (optional)

- Juice of 1 lime

- Ice cubes (optional)

Preparation:

- Combine kiwi slices, coconut milk, spinach leaves, honey or maple syrup (if using), and lime juice in a blender.

- Blend until smooth.

- Add ice cubes if you desired and blend again until smooth.

- Pour into a glass, garnish with a kiwi slice if desired, and serve immediately.

Green Goddess Brain Blend:

Ingredients:

- 1 cup spinach leaves

- 1/2 avocado

- 1/2 cup cucumber, chopped

- 1/2 cup pineapple chunks. (fresh or frozen)

- 1/2 cup coconut water or your almond milk

- 1 tablespoon chia seeds

- Ice cubes (optional)

Preparation:

● Place spinach leaves, avocado, chopped cucumber, pineapple chunks, coconut water or almond milk, and chia seeds in a blender.

● Blend until smooth and creamy.

● Add ice cubes if you desired and blend again until desired consistency is reached.

● Pour into a glass and enjoy this nourishing brain blend!

Broccoli Blueberry Brain Booster:

Ingredients:

- 1/2 cup broccoli florets

- 1/2 cup blueberries (fresh or frozen)

- 1/2 banana

- 1/2 cup plain Greek yogurt

- 1 tablespoon honey or maple syrup (optional)

- 1/2 cup unsweetened almond milk

- Ice cubes (optional)

Preparation:

• In a blender, combine broccoli florets, blueberries, banana, Greek yogurt, honey or maple syrup (if using), and almond milk.

• Blend until smooth and creamy.

• Add ice cubes if you desired and blend again until smooth.

• Pour into a glass and enjoy this brain-boosting smoothie!

Spirulina Banana Brain Booster:

Ingredients:

- 1 teaspoon spirulina powder

- 1/2 banana

- 1/2 cup spinach leaves

- 1/2 cup pineapple chunks. (fresh or frozen)

- 1/2 cup coconut water or your almond milk

- 1 tablespoon honey or maple syrup (optional)

- Ice cubes (optional)

Preparation:

- Combine spirulina powder, banana, spinach leaves, pineapple chunks, coconut water or almond milk, and honey or maple syrup (if using) in a blender.

- Blend until smooth and creamy.

- Add ice cubes if you desired and blend again until smooth.

- Pour into a glass and serve immediately for a refreshing brain booster!

Tropical Treasures for Mental Clarity

Mango Pineapple Paradise:

Ingredients:

- 1 cup mango chunks. (fresh or frozen)

- 1 cup pineapple chunks. (fresh or frozen)

- 1/2 banana

- 1/2 cup coconut water or coconut milk

- 1 tablespoon honey or maple syrup (optional)

- Ice cubes (optional)

Preparation:

• Combine mango chunks, pineapple chunks, banana, coconut water or coconut milk, and honey or maple syrup (if using) in a blender.

• Blend until smooth and creamy.

• Add ice cubes if you desired and blend again until desired consistency is reached.

• Pour into a glass and enjoy this tropical paradise smoothie!

Coconut Berry Breeze:

Ingredients:

- 1/2 cup mixed berries. (such as strawberries, blueberries, raspberries)

- 1/2 cup coconut milk

- 1/2 banana

- 1 tablespoon chia seeds

- 1 tablespoon shredded coconut (optional)

- Ice cubes (optional)

Preparation:

- In a blender, combine mixed berries, coconut milk, banana, and chia seeds.

- Blend until smooth.

- Add shredded coconut if using, and blend again briefly.

- Add ice cubes if you desired and blend until smooth.

- Pour into a glass, garnish with additional shredded coconut if desired, and enjoy this refreshing coconut berry breeze!

Papaya Passion Punch:

Ingredients:

- 1 cup papaya chunks. (fresh or frozen)

- 1/2 cup pineapple chunks. (fresh or frozen)

- 1/2 banana

- 1/2 cup orange juice

- 1 tablespoon honey or maple syrup (optional)

- Ice cubes (optional)

Preparation:

- Combine papaya chunks, pineapple chunks, banana, orange juice, and honey or maple syrup (if using) in a blender.

- Blend until smooth and creamy.

- Add ice cubes if you desired and blend again until desired consistency is reached.

- Pour into a glass, garnish with a slice of papaya or pineapple if desired, and enjoy this tropical punch!

Banana Turmeric Tonic:

Ingredients:

- 1/2 banana

- 1/2 cup mango chunks (fresh or frozen)

- 1/2 teaspoon turmeric powder

- 1/2 cup coconut water or your almond milk

- 1 tablespoon honey or maple syrup (optional)

- Ice cubes (optional)

Preparation:

• Place banana, mango chunks, turmeric powder, coconut water or almond milk, and honey or maple syrup (if using) in a blender.

• Blend until smooth.

• Add ice cubes if you desired and blend again until smooth.

• Pour into a glass, garnish with a sprinkle of turmeric if desired, and enjoy this refreshing turmeric tonic!

Pineapple Ginger Zinger:

Ingredients:

- 1 cup pineapple chunks. (fresh or frozen)

- 1/2 inch piece of fresh ginger, peel it and grated

- 1/2 banana

- 1/2 cup coconut water or the pineapple juice

- 1 tablespoon honey or maple syrup (optional)

- Ice cubes (optional)

Preparation:

- In a blender, combine pineapple chunks, grated ginger, banana, coconut water or pineapple juice, and honey or maple syrup (if using).

• Blend until smooth.

• Add ice cubes if you desired and blend again until smooth.

• Pour into a glass, garnish with a slice of pineapple or a sprinkle of grated ginger if desired, and enjoy this zesty pineapple ginger zinger!

Passionfruit Peach Brain Boost:

Ingredients:

• 1 passionfruit, pulp scooped out

• 1 ripe peach, pitted and chopped

- 1/2 cup coconut water or your almond milk

- 1/2 banana

- 1 tablespoon honey or maple syrup (optional)

- Ice cubes (optional)

Preparation:

- Combine passionfruit pulp, chopped peach, coconut water or almond milk, banana, and honey or maple syrup (if using) in a blender.

- Blend until smooth.

- Add ice cubes if you desired and blend again until smooth.

● Pour into a glass, garnish with a slice of peach or a passionfruit seed if desired, and enjoy this flavorful brain boost!

Guava Kiwi Brain Blend:

Ingredients:

● 1 guava, peeled and chopped

● 2 kiwis, peeled and chopped

● 1/2 banana

● 1/2 cup coconut water or kiwi juice

● 1 tablespoon honey or maple syrup (optional)

● Ice cubes (optional)

Preparation:

- Place chopped guava, kiwis, banana, coconut water or kiwi juice, and honey or maple syrup (if using) in a blender.

- Blend until smooth and creamy.

- Add ice cubes if desired and blend again until desired consistency is reached.

- Pour into a glass, garnish with a slice of kiwi or guava if desired, and enjoy this tropical brain blend!

Lychee Lime Brain Booster:

Ingredients:

- 1/2 cup lychee, peeled and pitted

- Juice of 1 lime

- 1/2 banana

- 1/2 cup coconut water or limeade

- 1 tablespoon honey or maple syrup (optional)

- Ice cubes (optional)

Preparation:

• Combine lychee, lime juice, banana, coconut water or limeade, and honey or maple syrup (if using) in a blender.

• Blend until smooth.

• Add ice cubes if you desired and blend again until smooth.

• Pour into a glass, garnish with a slice of lime or a lychee if desired, and enjoy this refreshing brain booster!

Nutty Nourishment for Cognitive Health

Almond Berry Brainwave:

Ingredients:

- 1/2 cup mixed berries. (such as strawberries, blueberries, raspberries)

- 1/2 banana

- 1 tablespoon almond butter

- 1/2 cup almond milk

- 1 tablespoon honey or maple syrup (optional)

- Ice cubes (optional)

Preparation:

- In a blender, combine mixed berries, banana, almond butter, almond milk, and honey or maple syrup (if using).

- Blend until smooth.

- Add ice cubes if desired and blend again until desired consistency is reached.

- Pour into a glass, garnish with a few whole berries if desired, and enjoy this almond berry brainwave!

Walnut Banana Bonanza:

Ingredients:

- 1/2 banana

- 1/4 cup walnuts

- 1/2 cup Greek yogurt

- 1/2 cup milk (dairy or plant-based)

- 1 tablespoon honey or maple syrup (optional)

Ice cubes (optional)

Preparation:

- Place banana, walnuts, Greek yogurt, milk, and honey or maple syrup (if using) in a blender.

- Blend until smooth.

- Add ice cubes if you desired and blend again until smooth.

- Pour into a glass, garnish with a sprinkle of chopped walnuts if desired, and enjoy this walnut banana bonanza!

Peanut Butter Power Smoothie:

Ingredients:

- 1 tablespoon peanut butter

- 1/2 banana

- 1/2 cup spinach leaves

- 1/2 cup almond milk

- 1 tablespoon honey or maple syrup (optional)

- Ice cubes (optional)

Preparation:

- In a blender, combine peanut butter, banana, spinach leaves, almond milk, and honey or maple syrup (if using).

- Blend until smooth.

- Add ice cubes if you desired and blend again until smooth.

- Pour into a glass, garnish with a drizzle of peanut butter if desired, and enjoy this peanut butter power smoothie!

Hazelnut Chocolate Cognition Elixir:

Ingredients:

- 1 tablespoon hazelnut spread (such as Nutella)

- 1/2 banana

- 1 tablespoon cocoa powder

- 1/2 cup milk (dairy or plant-based)

- 1 tablespoon honey or maple syrup (optional)

- Ice cubes (optional)

Preparation:

- Combine hazelnut spread, banana, cocoa powder, milk, and honey or maple syrup (if using) in a blender.

- Blend until smooth.

- Add ice cubes if you desired and blend again until smooth.

- Pour into a glass, garnish with a sprinkle of cocoa powder if desired, and enjoy this indulgent hazelnut chocolate cognition elixir!

Cashew Date Brain Boost:

Ingredients:

- 1/4 cup cashews

- 2-3 pitted dates

- 1/2 banana

- 1/2 cup almond milk

- 1 tablespoon honey or maple syrup (optional)

- Ice cubes (optional)

Preparation:

- In a blender, combine cashews, dates, banana, almond milk, and honey or maple syrup (if using).

- Blend until smooth.

- Add ice cubes if you desired and blend again until smooth.

- Pour into a glass, garnish with a slice of date if desired, and enjoy this nourishing cashew date brain boost!

Pecan Pie Brain Blend:

Ingredients:

- 1/4 cup pecans

- 1/2 banana

- 1/4 teaspoon cinnamon

- 1/2 cup Greek yogurt

- 1/2 cup milk (dairy or plant-based)

- 1 tablespoon honey or maple syrup (optional)

- Ice cubes (optional)

Preparation:

- Combine pecans, banana, cinnamon, Greek yogurt, milk, and honey or maple syrup (if using) in a blender.

- Blend until smooth.

- Add ice cubes if you desired and blend again until smooth.

- Pour into a glass, garnish with a sprinkle of cinnamon if desired, and enjoy this pecan pie brain blend!

Macadamia Mango Brain Booster:

Ingredients:

- 1/4 cup macadamia nuts

- 1/2 cup mango chunks (fresh or frozen)

- 1/2 banana

- 1/2 cup coconut milk

- 1 tablespoon honey or maple syrup (optional)

- Ice cubes (optional)

Preparation:

- Place macadamia nuts, mango chunks, banana, coconut milk, and honey or maple syrup (if using) in a blender.

- Blend until smooth and creamy.

- Add ice cubes if desired and blend again until desired consistency is reached.

- Pour into a glass, garnish with a slice of mango if desired, and enjoy this tropical macadamia mango brain booster!

Pistachio Berry Brain Blast:

Ingredients:

- 1/4 cup shelled pistachios

- 1/2 cup mixed berries. (such as strawberries, blueberries, raspberries)

- 1/2 banana

- 1/2 cup almond milk

- 1 tablespoon honey or maple syrup (optional)

- Ice cubes (optional)

Preparation:

• In a blender, combine pistachios, mixed berries, banana, almond milk, and honey or maple syrup (if using).

• Blend until smooth.

• Add ice cubes if you desired and blend again until smooth.

• Pour into a glass, garnish with a few crushed pistachios if desired, and enjoy this pistachio berry brain blast!

Superfood Sips for Brain Function

Acai Berry Brainwave:

Ingredients:

- 1/2 cup frozen acai berries

- 1/2 banana

- 1/2 cup mixed berries. (such as strawberries, blueberries, raspberries)

- 1/2 cup almond milk

- 1 tablespoon honey or maple syrup (optional)

- Ice cubes (optional)

Preparation:

• In a blender, combine frozen acai berries, banana, mixed berries, almond milk, and honey or maple syrup (if using).

• Blend until smooth.

• Add ice cubes if you desired and blend again until smooth.

• Pour into a glass, garnish with a few acai berries if desired, and enjoy this acai berry brainwave!

Chia Seed Brain Booster:

Ingredients:

- 1 tablespoon chia seeds

- 1/2 cup mixed berries. (such as strawberries, blueberries, raspberries)

- 1/2 banana

- 1/2 cup spinach leaves

- 1/2 cup almond milk

- 1 tablespoon honey or maple syrup (optional)

- Ice cubes (optional)

Preparation:

- In a blender, combine chia seeds, mixed berries, banana, spinach leaves, almond milk, and honey or maple syrup (if using).

• Blend until smooth.

• Add ice cubes if you desired and blend again until smooth.

• Pour into a glass, garnish with a sprinkle of chia seeds if desired, and enjoy this chia seed brain booster!

Flaxseed Berry Blast:

Ingredients:

• 1 tablespoon ground flaxseeds

• 1/2 cup mixed berries. (such as strawberries, blueberries, raspberries)

• 1/2 banana

- 1/2 cup Greek yogurt

- 1/2 cup almond milk

- 1 tablespoon honey or maple syrup (optional)

- Ice cubes (optional)

Preparation:

- Combine ground flaxseeds, mixed berries, banana, Greek yogurt, almond milk, and honey or maple syrup (if using) in a blender.

- Blend until smooth.

- Add ice cubes if you desired and blend again until smooth.

- Pour into a glass, garnish with a sprinkle of ground flaxseeds if desired, and enjoy this flaxseed berry blast!

Hemp Heart Mind Mixer:

Ingredients:

- 1 tablespoon hemp hearts

- 1/2 cup mixed berries. (such as strawberries, blueberries, raspberries)

- 1/2 banana

- 1/2 cup spinach leaves

- 1/2 cup almond milk

- 1 tablespoon honey or maple syrup (optional)

- Ice cubes (optional)

Preparation:

• In a blender, combine hemp hearts, mixed berries, banana, spinach leaves, almond milk, and honey or maple syrup (if using).

• Blend until smooth.

• Add ice cubes if you desired and blend again until smooth.

• Pour into a glass, garnish with a sprinkle of hemp hearts if desired, and enjoy this hemp heart mind mixer!

Quinoa Blueberry Brilliance:

Ingredients:

- 1/4 cup cooked quinoa, cooled

- 1/2 cup mixed berries. (such as strawberries, blueberries, raspberries)

- 1/2 banana

- 1/2 cup Greek yogurt

- 1/2 cup almond milk

- 1 tablespoon honey or maple syrup (optional)

- Ice cubes (optional)

Preparation:

• In a blender, combine cooked quinoa, mixed berries, banana, Greek yogurt, almond milk, and honey or maple syrup (if using).

• Blend until smooth.

• Add ice cubes if you desired and blend again until smooth.

• Pour into a glass, garnish with a few cooked quinoa grains if desired, and enjoy this quinoa blueberry brilliance!

Spirulina Berry Brain Boost:

Ingredients:

- 1 teaspoon spirulina powder

- 1/2 cup mixed berries. (such as strawberries, blueberries, raspberries)

- 1/2 banana

- 1/2 cup spinach leaves

- 1/2 cup almond milk

- 1 tablespoon honey or maple syrup (optional)

- Ice cubes (optional)

Preparation:

• In a blender, combine spirulina powder, mixed berries, banana, spinach leaves, almond milk, and honey or maple syrup (if using).

• Blend until smooth.

• Add ice cubes if you desired and blend again until smooth.

• Pour into a glass, garnish with a sprinkle of spirulina powder if desired, and enjoy this spirulina berry brain boost!

Wheatgrass Green Goddess Smoothie:

Ingredients:

- 1 tablespoon wheatgrass powder

- 1/2 cup mixed berries. (such as strawberries, blueberries, raspberries)

- 1/2 banana

- 1/2 cup spinach leaves

1/2 cup coconut water

- 1 tablespoon honey or maple syrup (optional)

- Ice cubes (optional)

Preparation:

- Combine wheatgrass powder, mixed berries, banana, spinach leaves, coconut water, and honey or maple syrup (if using) in a blender.

- Blend until smooth.

- Add ice cubes if you desired and blend again until smooth.

- Pour into a glass, garnish with a sprinkle of wheatgrass powder if desired, and enjoy this wheatgrass green goddess smoothie!

Maca Root Mango Mind Mix:

Ingredients:

- 1 teaspoon maca root powder

- 1/2 cup mango chunks (fresh or frozen)

- 1/2 banana

- 1/2 cup Greek yogurt

- 1/2 cup almond milk

- 1 tablespoon honey or maple syrup (optional)

- Ice cubes (optional)

Preparation:

• Place maca root powder, mango chunks, banana, Greek yogurt, almond milk, and honey or maple syrup (if using) in a blender.

• Blend until smooth.

• Add ice cubes if you desired and blend again until smooth.

• Pour into a glass, garnish with a sprinkle of maca root powder if desired, and enjoy this maca root mango mind mix!

Spice Infusions for Cognitive Enhancement

Turmeric Ginger Golden Blend:

Ingredients:

- 1 teaspoon ground turmeric

- 1 teaspoon grated fresh ginger

- 1/2 banana

- 1/2 cup pineapple chunks. (fresh or frozen)

- 1/2 cup Greek yogurt

- 1/2 cup almond milk

- 1 tablespoon honey or maple syrup (optional)

• Ice cubes (optional)

Preparation:

• Place ground turmeric, grated fresh ginger, banana, pineapple chunks, Greek yogurt, almond milk, and honey or maple syrup (if using) in a blender.

• Blend until smooth.

• Add ice cubes if you desired and blend again until smooth.

• Pour into a glass, garnish with a sprinkle of ground turmeric if desired, and enjoy this turmeric ginger golden blend!

Cinnamon Apple Cognitive Cooler:

Ingredients:

- 1/2 teaspoon ground cinnamon

- 1/2 apple, cored and chopped

- 1/2 banana

- 1/2 cup spinach leaves

- 1/2 cup almond milk

- 1 tablespoon honey or maple syrup (optional)

- Ice cubes (optional)

Preparation:

- Combine ground cinnamon, apple chunks, banana, spinach leaves, almond milk, and honey or maple syrup (if using) in a blender.

- Blend until smooth.

- Add ice cubes if you desired and blend again until smooth.

- Pour into a glass, garnish with a sprinkle of ground cinnamon if desired, and enjoy this cinnamon apple cognitive cooler!

Cardamom Banana Brain Booster:

Ingredients:

- 1/4 teaspoon ground cardamom

- 1/2 banana

- 1/2 cup mixed berries. (such as strawberries, blueberries, raspberries)

- 1/2 cup Greek yogurt

- 1/2 cup almond milk

- 1 tablespoon honey or maple syrup (optional)

- Ice cubes (optional)

Preparation:

- In a blender, combine ground cardamom, banana, mixed berries, Greek yogurt, almond milk, and honey or maple syrup (if using).

- Blend until smooth.

- Add ice cubes if you desired and blend again until smooth.

- Pour into a glass, garnish with a sprinkle of ground cardamom if desired, and enjoy this cardamom banana brain booster!

Ginger Berry Brain Fuel:

Ingredients:

- 1 teaspoon grated fresh ginger

- 1/2 cup mixed berries. (such as strawberries, blueberries, raspberries)

- 1/2 banana

- 1/2 cup spinach leaves

- 1/2 cup almond milk

- 1 tablespoon honey or maple syrup (optional)

- Ice cubes (optional)

Preparation:

- Combine grated fresh ginger, mixed berries, banana, spinach leaves, almond milk, and honey or maple syrup (if using) in a blender.

- Blend until smooth.

- Add ice cubes if you desired and blend again until smooth.

- Pour into a glass, garnish with a slice of fresh ginger if desired, and enjoy this ginger berry brain fuel!

Cayenne Mango Mental Energizer:

Ingredients:

- 1/4 teaspoon ground cayenne pepper

- 1/2 cup mango chunks (fresh or frozen)

- 1/2 banana

- 1/2 cup Greek yogurt

- 1/2 cup almond milk

- 1 tablespoon honey or maple syrup (optional)

- Ice cubes (optional)

Preparation:

• In a blender, combine ground cayenne pepper, mango chunks, banana, Greek yogurt, almond milk, and honey or maple syrup (if using).

• Blend until smooth.

• Add ice cubes if you desired and blend again until smooth.

• Pour into a glass, garnish with a sprinkle of ground cayenne pepper if desired, and enjoy this cayenne mango mental energizer!

Black Pepper Blueberry Brain Blend:

Ingredients:

- 1/4 teaspoon ground black pepper

- 1/2 cup blueberries (fresh or frozen)

- 1/2 banana

- 1/2 cup spinach leaves

- 1/2 cup almond milk

- 1 tablespoon honey or maple syrup (optional)

- Ice cubes (optional)

Preparation:

- Combine ground black pepper, blueberries, banana, spinach leaves, almond milk, and honey or maple syrup (if using) in a blender.

- Blend until smooth.

- Add ice cubes if you desired and blend again until smooth.

- Pour into a glass, garnish with a sprinkle of ground black pepper if desired, and enjoy this black pepper blueberry brain blend!

Clove Cranberry Cognitive Cooler:

Ingredients:

- 1/4 teaspoon ground cloves

- 1/2 cup cranberries (fresh or frozen)

- 1/2 banana

- 1/2 cup Greek yogurt

- 1/2 cup almond milk

- 1 tablespoon honey or maple syrup (optional)

- Ice cubes (optional)

Preparation:

- In a blender, combine ground cloves, cranberries, banana, Greek yogurt, almond milk, and honey or maple syrup (if using).

- Blend until smooth.

- Add ice cubes if you desired and blend again until smooth.

- Pour into a glass, garnish with a sprinkle of ground cloves if desired, and enjoy this clove cranberry cognitive cooler!

Nutmeg Nectarine Brain Booster:

Ingredients:

- 1/4 teaspoon ground nutmeg

- 1/2 nectarine, pitted and chopped

- 1/2 banana

- 1/2 cup spinach leaves

- 1/2 cup almond milk

- 1 tablespoon honey or maple syrup (optional)

- Ice cubes (optional)

Preparation:

- Combine ground nutmeg, chopped nectarine, banana, spinach leaves, almond milk, and honey or maple syrup (if using) in a blender.

- Blend until smooth.

- Add ice cubes if you desired and blend again until smooth.

- Pour into a glass, garnish with a sprinkle of ground nutmeg if desired, enjoy.

Sweet and Savory Smoothies for Cognitive Wellness

Avocado Chocolate Dream:

Ingredients:

- 1/2 ripe avocado

- 1 tablespoon cocoa powder

- 1 tablespoon honey or maple syrup

- 1/2 cup almond milk

- 1/2 banana

- Ice cubes (optional)

Preparation:

- Scoop out the flesh of your avocado and place it in the blender.

- Add cocoa powder, honey or maple syrup, almond milk, and banana to the blender.

- Blend until smooth.

- Add ice cubes if you desired and blend again until smooth.

- Pour into a glass and enjoy this creamy avocado chocolate dream!

Sweet Potato Pie Power Smoothie:

Ingredients:

- 1/2 cup cooked and mashed sweet potato

- 1/2 cup Greek yogurt

- 1/2 banana

- 1/4 teaspoon ground cinnamon

- 1 tablespoon honey or maple syrup

- 1/2 cup almond milk

- Ice cubes (optional)

Preparation:

- In a blender, combine mashed sweet potato, Greek yogurt, banana, ground cinnamon, honey or maple syrup, and almond milk.

- Blend until smooth.

- Add ice cubes if you desired and blend again until smooth.

- Pour into a glass and enjoy this sweet potato pie power smoothie!

Beet Berry Brain Boost:

Ingredients:

- 1/2 cooked beetroot, peeled and chopped

- 1/2 cup mixed berries. (such as strawberries, blueberries, raspberries)

- 1/2 banana

- 1/2 cup spinach leaves

- 1/2 cup almond milk

- 1 tablespoon honey or maple syrup

- Ice cubes (optional)

Preparation:

• Place cooked beetroot, mixed berries, banana, spinach leaves, almond milk, and honey or maple syrup in a blender.

• Blend until smooth.

• Add ice cubes if you desired and blend again until smooth.

• Pour into a glass and enjoy this vibrant beet berry brain boost!

Carrot Cake Cognition Elixir:

Ingredients:

- 1/2 cup cooked and mashed carrot

- 1/2 cup Greek yogurt

- 1/4 teaspoon ground nutmeg

- 1 tablespoon honey or maple syrup

- 1/2 cup almond milk

- Ice cubes (optional)

Preparation:

- In a blender, combine mashed carrot, Greek yogurt, ground nutmeg, honey or maple syrup, and almond milk.

- Blend until smooth.

- Add ice cubes if you desired and blend again until smooth.

- Pour into a glass and enjoy this carrot cake cognition elixir!

Tomato Basil Brain Booster:

Ingredients:

- 1/2 cup cherry tomatoes

- 1/4 cup fresh basil leaves

- 1/2 cup cucumber, chopped

- 1/2 avocado

- 1/2 cup spinach leaves

- 1/2 cup almond milk

- Juice of 1/2 lemon

- Salt and pepper to taste

- Ice cubes (optional)

Preparation:

- In a blender, combine cherry tomatoes, basil leaves, chopped cucumber, avocado, spinach leaves, almond milk, lemon juice, salt, and pepper.

- Blend until smooth.

- Add ice cubes if you desired and blend again until smooth.

- Pour into a glass and enjoy this refreshing tomato basil brain booster!

Pumpkin Spice Brain Blend:

Ingredients:

- 1/2 cup canned pumpkin puree

- 1/2 banana

- 1/4 teaspoon ground cinnamon

- 1/4 teaspoon ground nutmeg

- 1 tablespoon honey or maple syrup

- 1/2 cup almond milk

- Ice cubes (optional)

Preparation:

• In a blender, combine pumpkin puree, banana, ground cinnamon, ground nutmeg, honey or maple syrup, and almond milk.

• Blend until smooth.

• Add ice cubes if you desired and blend again until smooth.

• Pour into a glass and enjoy this cozy pumpkin spice brain blend!

Spinach Banana Brain Booster:

Ingredients:

- 1/2 banana

- 1/2 cup spinach leaves

- 1/2 cup Greek yogurt

- 1 tablespoon almond butter

- 1 tablespoon honey or maple syrup

- 1/2 cup almond milk

- Ice cubes (optional)

Preparation:

- In a blender, combine banana, spinach leaves, Greek yogurt, almond butter, honey or maple syrup, and almond milk.

- Blend until smooth.

- Add ice cubes if you desired and blend again until smooth.

- Pour into a glass and enjoy this nutrient-packed spinach banana brain booster!

Chickpea Chocolate Brain Booster:

Ingredients:

- 1/2 cup cooked chickpeas. (canned is fine)

- 1 tablespoon cocoa powder

- 1 tablespoon honey or maple syrup

- 1/2 cup almond milk

- 1/2 banana

- Ice cubes (optional)

Preparation:

- Place cooked chickpeas, cocoa powder, honey or maple syrup, almond milk, and banana in a blender.

- Blend until smooth.

- Add ice cubes if you desired and blend again until smooth.

- Pour into a glass and enjoy this unique chickpea chocolate brain booster!

Hydration Blends for Brain Hygiene

Coconut Water Blueberry Blast:

Ingredients:

- 1/2 cup coconut water

- 1/2 cup blueberries

- 1/2 banana

- 1/2 cup spinach leaves

- 1 tablespoon honey or maple syrup

- Ice cubes (optional)

Preparation:

• In a blender, combine coconut water, blueberries, banana, spinach leaves, and honey or maple syrup.

• Blend until smooth.

• Add ice cubes if you desired and blend again until smooth.

• Pour into a glass and enjoy this refreshing coconut water blueberry blast!

Cucumber Celery Brain Cleanse:

Ingredients:

- 1/2 cucumber, chopped

- 2 celery stalks, chopped

- 1/2 cup spinach leaves

- 1/2 cup coconut water

- Juice of 1/2 lemon

- Small piece of ginger (optional)

- Ice cubes (optional)

Preparation:

- Place chopped cucumber, celery stalks, spinach leaves, coconut water, lemon juice, and ginger (if using) in a blender.

- Blend until smooth.

- Add ice cubes if you desired and blend again until smooth.

- Pour into a glass and enjoy this cleansing cucumber celery brain cleanse!

Watermelon Mint Mind Refresher:

Ingredients:

- 1 cup diced watermelon

- 1 tablespoon fresh mint leaves

- 1/2 cup coconut water

- Juice of 1/2 lime

- 1 tablespoon honey or maple syrup

- Ice cubes (optional)

Preparation:

- In a blender, combine diced watermelon, fresh mint leaves, coconut water, lime juice, and honey or maple syrup.

- Blend until smooth.

- Add ice cubes if you desired and blend again until smooth.

- Pour into a glass and enjoy this revitalizing watermelon mint mind refresher!

Lemon Lime Hydration Infusion:

Ingredients:

- Juice of 1 lemon

- Juice of 1 lime

- 1 tablespoon honey or maple syrup

- 1/2 cup coconut water

- 1/2 cup cold water

- Ice cubes (optional)

Preparation:

- In a blender, combine lemon juice, lime juice, honey or maple syrup, coconut water, and cold water.

- Blend until well combined.

- Add ice cubes if you desired and blend again until smooth.

- Pour into a glass and enjoy this hydrating lemon lime infusion!

Green Tea Berry Brainwash:

Ingredients:

- 1/2 cup brewed green tea, cooled

- 1/2 cup mixed berries. (such as strawberries, blueberries, raspberries)

- 1/2 banana

- 1 tablespoon honey or maple syrup

- 1/2 cup spinach leaves

- Ice cubes (optional)

Preparation:

- In a blender, combine brewed green tea, mixed berries, banana, honey or maple syrup, and spinach leaves.

- Blend until smooth.

- Add ice cubes if you desired and blend again until smooth.

- Pour into a glass and enjoy this antioxidant-rich green tea berry brainwash!

Cranberry Cucumber Brain Boost:

Ingredients:

- 1/2 cup cranberries (fresh or frozen)

- 1/2 cucumber, chopped

- 1/2 cup coconut water

- Juice of 1/2 lemon

- 1 tablespoon honey or maple syrup

- Ice cubes (optional)

Preparation:

- Place cranberries, chopped cucumber, coconut water, lemon juice, and honey or maple syrup in a blender.

- Blend until smooth.

- Add ice cubes if you desired and blend again until smooth.

- Pour into a glass and enjoy this refreshing cranberry cucumber brain boost!

Aloe Vera Brain Booster:

Ingredients:

- 1 tablespoon aloe vera gel. (from a fresh aloe vera leaf)

- 1/2 cup coconut water

- 1/2 cup pineapple chunks

- 1/2 cup spinach leaves

- 1 tablespoon honey or maple syrup

- Ice cubes (optional)

Preparation:

- In a blender, combine aloe vera gel, coconut water, pineapple chunks, spinach leaves, and honey or maple syrup.

- Blend until smooth.

- Add ice cubes if you desired and blend again until smooth.

- Pour into a glass and enjoy this hydrating aloe vera brain booster!

Herbal Infusion Brain Blend:

Ingredients:

- 1/2 cup herbal infusion. (such as chamomile, peppermint, or ginger tea), cooled

- 1/2 cup mixed berries. (such as strawberries, blueberries, raspberries)

- 1/2 banana

- 1 tablespoon honey or maple syrup

- 1/2 cup spinach leaves

- Ice cubes (optional)

Preparation:

• In a blender, combine herbal infusion, mixed berries, banana, honey or maple syrup, and spinach leaves.

• Blend until smooth.

• Add ice cubes if you desired and blend again until smooth.

• Pour into a glass and enjoy this soothing herbal infusion brain blend!

Conclusion

MIND Diet Smoothie Recipes Cookbook offers a delicious and nutritious way to support cognitive wellness and brain health. By incorporating nutrient-rich ingredients and delicious flavors into smoothie recipes, this cookbook provides a convenient and enjoyable way to nourish the mind and body.

Whether you're looking to boost your cognitive function, improve memory and focus, or simply enjoy a refreshing and satisfying beverage, the recipes in this cookbook are designed to help you achieve your wellness goals.

With a focus on wholesome ingredients and simple preparation instructions, these smoothies can easily be integrated into your daily routine.

Here's to a healthier and happier you with each sip of these brain-boosting smoothies!